Yan d'Albert

SUFI HEALING

Book

They draw on a tradition that goes back thousands of years. Their motivation of healing is a vocation and comes deep from the heart. Their motto is:

„For every illness, there's a remedy"

From the content:

- *What does Sufi mean?*

- *Breath and mindfulness*

- *Preferred healing food and application*

- *The healing water*

The author

`Abd al-Malik Dildar* Yan d'Albert (*1958 in Augsburg, Germany) is a musician, music and Sufi teacher, author of books, and publisher. He is the founder and head of MUSIKHAUS ALBERT which includes school, shop, music production & edition in Bergisch Gladbach, near Cologne. He is also a representative of the SUFI MOVEMENT Germany and initiator of SUFI WAY OF HEART AND HEALING.

Yan d'Albert

SUFI HEALING

including miraculous thoughts,
prayers and meditations
for protection and healing

editionsol

The informations and recommendations presented here have been reviewed to the best knowledge and belief, nevertheless, the author and publisher does not take any liability for any direct or indirect damages resulting from the use of the applications presented here. In any case, please observe the limits of self-treatment and make use of a professional diagnosis and therapy by medical or natural help in the event of disease symptoms.

English edition: SUFI HEALING
German original edition: DIE HEILKUNST DER SUFIS.
English reader: Karin Bolinius, Yan d'Albert

1st English edition 2018 edition**sol**
2nd English edition 2021 edition**sol**
CreateSpace ISBN: 9781542417259

Content

> *The natural desire of every soul is to live; to have a life of perfect health; to make the best of one's coming into this world.*
> Hazrat Inayat-Khan

> *And when I am sick, He heals me.*
> Holy Quran, Sura al-Schu´ara´ (The Poets), Sura 26:80

Preface

Dear reader, Sisters & Brothers all over the world!

The world needs cure, "our" planet earth needs healing! Urgently. More than ever. How long menhood wants to hesitate to apply the right medicine? How long menhood will ignore its Creator? He Alone is the All-Healer, al-Shâfi, and the Capable of anything, al-Kâfi. To listen to Him, to believe in Him and to do His will is the absolute requirement for His Mercy of giving healing.

I have the great pleasure and honour to introduce you to the English version of my German book DIE HEILKUNST DER SUFIS (THE SUFI ART OF HEALING). The Prophet – peace and blessings be upon him – said: "**Allâh** has not sent down a disease except that He sent down its cure."

I wish you maximum benefits and blessings with this book. May **Allâh**, the All-Healing, present you abundantly with healing and health, inscha **Allâh**!

With all my heart

`Abd al-Malik Dildar Yan d'Albert,
Bergisch Gladbach, AH 1443 and 2021 CE

1

The diversity of Sufi healing

They are mystics, messengers and wonder workers, saints and healers in the name and on behalf of God. They draw on a tradition that goes back thousands of years. Their motivation of healing is a vocation and comes deep from the heart. Because with their healing methods, they prefer to work secretly, voluntarily, and without payment, not to be named or to be honored. Their motto is: „For every illness there's a remedy". Here they do not only use physical remedies, but also mental and emotional ones. Faith is first and foremost the basis and condition for a healing process. The cultivation of certain virtues like thankfulness, forgiveness, beneficence, etc. is also helpful. In the prayer and healing circles of the Sufis, one can feel the deep power of word and prayer. In order to stay or to become healthy, the Sufis use special healing food and oils. They know the secrets of the magic of words and numbers and they create special formulas and amulets for healing purposes. They also attach great importance to fasting, they cultivate music, dance, and humour. The Sufi art of healing must only be considered holistically; its nature is versatile and rich.

The Sufi Message does not give a new law. It awakens the spirit of brotherhood in humanity, which is accompanied by tolerance on the part of each towards the religion of the other, and the general willingness to forgive the faults of the others. It teaches thoughtfulness and consideration to create and maintain a life in harmony; it also teaches to serve and make oneself truly useful, which alone can make life in the world fruitful and in which lies the satisfaction of every soul.
Hazrat Inayat Khan

2

What does „Sufi" mean?

What does this word actually mean? S U F I ..., it sounds like a mysterious magic word, a subtle mantra. Relating to the etymology of the term, there are different and unclear definitions: On the basis of the Arabic root **sûf**, it has the meaning "wool", "purity", and "transparency". Early mystics such as *John the Baptist* or *Jesus of Nazareth* (peace be with them) wore woolen garments and they also rank among the Sufis. "Sufiya" is the "one chosen as intimate friend (of God)". They are also said to be the successors of the disciples, who once lived in the forecourt of the prophet *Muhammad*. With the term "Sufi" – as far as the word is known – most people associate a picture of dancing, oriental dervishes with white clothes and high hats. But only referred to this, it remains a cliché. After all, since the birth of Sufi communities in the beginning of the first millennium after Christ, significantly more than 100 Sufi orders have formed, so-called *turuq*, which almost all still exist until today. The members may differ in appearance, but internal intention and orientation of all Sufis are the same: **Divine Wisdom & Love.** This is also the shortest possible definition of "Sufism". Its roots can be found in all traditions and can be traced back to the creation of man.

An old allegory is as follows:

> The seed of Sufism
> was sown by *Adam*,
> came to growth in the time of *Noah*,
> developed under *Abraham*,
> began to mature during *Moses*
> reached its full maturity with *Jesus*
> and produced the pure wine through *Muhammad*
> *(peace be with all of them).*

One of the central personalities of the Sufi tradition is the Indian musician and mystic *Hazrat Inayat-Khan* (1882-1927). He is the first representative of a universal Sufism, which towers over religions and limits. We owe it to this great master, musician, and mystic, that the Sufi message gained a large distribution in a universal spirituality in the beginning of the 20th century. His *"Sufi Message"* in 14 volumes is addressed to the Western world and is divided into lectures, poems and aphorisms. This literary work includes all spiritual areas of life and mystic teachings of the Sufi tradition. It contains precious wisdoms of fascinating beauty and loving heart. The trends resulting from the work of *Inayat Khan, Sufi Order, Sufi Movement, Sufi Way,* more specifically *Inayati Order,* build spiritual "acupoints" worldwide and are open to all interested persons. Many seekers, by turning their attention to the Sufi path and in accordance with an initiation from a teacher or *Shaikh,* have found their individual pathway and aim in life, love, harmony, and beauty, healing, health, and peace.

Due to the acute global problems of humanity, the Sufi message is more important than ever. By constantly undergoing a transformation, the orders and movements could remain the same open and authentic, until today. If this would not be the case, dogmatism and stagnation would be the rule.

Sufis are not only the mystics of Islam but in a universal sense also the mystical representatives of all religions and spiritual traditions. They have always been the once to wake people up and admonishers of their time. They are the ones who love and praise the truth and make service to others close to their hearts.

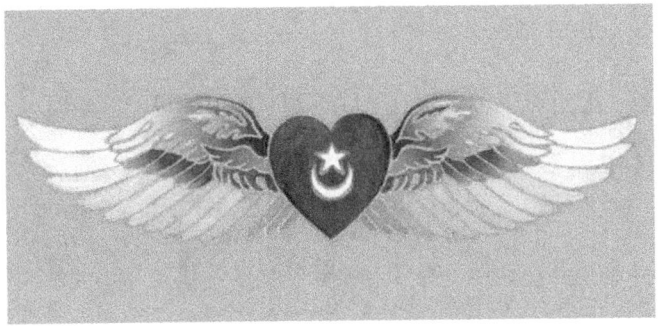

The heart with wings, star and crescent moon, symbol of some Sufi orders.

3

The Sufi healing orders

In all Sufi orders of whatever religious or philosophic orientation or school, it is a major priority to help sick and suffering people. Within there are numerous experienced medical professionals, doctors, therapists and healers world wide. Below I introduce to you some of the most active and famous ones:

The ancient healing tradition of the Chishti Order / Spiritual Healing Treatment

A wonderful example is the Sufi order of the *Chishti,* an Indian *tariqa*, who's members intensively dedicate themselves to the healing of sick people for over 800 years. Not a meeting goes by without offering assistance for needy people and enclosing them in prayers.

Under the spiritual command of *Sheikh Mu'in al-Din Chishti,* also known as *Hazrat Khwaja Gharib Nawaz,* the most famous Islamic mystic and Sufi Sheikh of the *Chishti Order,* Spiritual Healing Treatment is always in service of people, under the guidance of *Chief Moallim Gaddinashin (Peer Sahab) Syed Imran Chishty.* They provide free spiritual treatment for all kind of problems and diseases. According to statement not only spiritual healing (prayers, zikr, du'as) is practiced but also contact healing. " The method of contact healing is also used in this spiritual healing. It is so straightforward Magic of Healing. The technique involves cleansing the patient's aura and sending

spiritual energy into his/her body and the area of discomfort by visualization and physical contact."
Source: www.taweezdargahajmer.com

For more information see:
www.taweezdargahajmer.com
www.chishti.org
www.khwajagharibnawaz.com

The Sufi Healing Order / Raphaelite Work

The Sufi Healing Order is an international organization dedicated to nurturing and developing spiritual healing in our time. In many cities round the world, groups with healing circles regularly come together. All people are welcome to what they offer. Within this order, the so called *Raphaelite Work* (www.raphaelite.work) of the network of the same name is active and comprises three main activities: The Raphaelite Work Hands-on Healing Session, The Raphaelite Work One-to-One Healing Session and The Raphaelite Work Retreat.

Healing and transformation through presence, breath and touch

The Raphaelite work is an approach to healing, transformation, and discovery that supports one in living life more fully. Firmly rooted in Sufism and other wisdom traditions, it is enriched with insights from modern psychology, scientific research, and clinical practice. At the heart of the Raphaelite Work, named for the Archangel Raphael, angel of healing and science, is an understanding that there are many ways to experience life. This Work encourages one to be ever more present to, and familiar with, the unique languages of the physical, mental, emotional, moral, and spiritual aspects of self. When the intelligences of these different bodies are allowed to manifest in an atmosphere that is gentle, non-directive, and non-judgmental, a healing takes place which is both restorative and transformative.

The Raphaelite Work Hands-on Healing Session

The Raphaelite Work healing session begins with a pre-session interview, orienting both the client and the practitioner to a place in which to begin the session. While the client is fully dressed and lying on a massage table or a futon on the floor, the Raphaelite Work practitioner gently places his/her hands on specific points of the client's body relating to the elements: earth, water, fire, air, and ether. These points are used to enable a discussion of any sensations, thoughts or feelings that might arise. The Hands-on Healing session is followed by a post-session interview; this time is spent on helping to integrate the information from the five domains, on observing how the energy is flowing, and on recognizing whatever changes may have occurred within the domains.

The Raphaelite Work One-to-One Healing Session

The client and the One-to-One facilitator begin a discussion centering on the client's relationship to her/his experiences of the five domains. Through a healing presence in a One-to-One session, the client will find clarity developing in her/his understanding of self and her/his relationship to others. The One-to-One facilitator, listening from her/his heart, using love and compassion, and allowing the client to feel at ease, will use breath, and inquiry, resulting in a gentle, non-directive, non-judgmental atmosphere. The facilitator does not give advice, share opinions, or become personally involved in the client's process.

The Raphaelite Work Retreat

With the guidance of a Raphaelite Work Retreat guide, the Raphaelite Retreat offers time and space to be with oneself, exploring the language and the flow of energies in the five domains in depth. While on retreat, one leaves the day-to-day activities of life behind, and is supported in turning one's attention inward. The Raphaelite Work Retreat deepens and clarifies the relationship with one's self and life, offering a greater clarity in dealing with everyday problems. Through using practices of breath, and presence, and in working within the five domains, a new sense of self develops, and a new feeling of joy may emerge. A five day retreat is recommended; however, retreats of shorter duration may be arranged.

For further information see:
www.sufihealingorder.org
www.raphaelite.work

4

Healing all and everywhere

Healing practices naturally are limited not only to human beings. Also animals, plants, places, landscapes, cities, countries … yeahh, the whole world can be integrated in healing processes. Just like with humans, in whose cells and fields events and experienced are saved, this is also the case with buildings and plots. But often there is no harmony and peace because of the presence of bad and unresolved energies.

Geomancy is the science of healing the earth, the art to experience energy fields of the earth and to use the knowledge creatively. Our Celtic-Germanic ancestors have been great masters of the *geomancy*. "Our" earth is a living body, sensitive, sensible and vulnerable. Too often it was disturbed and partially destroyed by human interventions. "Mother Earth" is suffering on the following of crimes, suicides, wars etc. Special places bear special healing energies. Graves of saints have these healing and illuminating effects. Or let's think of the Holy City *Mecca* with its *Zamzam* well and its healing water.

What could be better, as servant of **Allâh**, the Almighty and His creation, than to use Holy Words, Prayers, Mantras, Wazifas and Du'as as remedy for all and everywhere. As a wonderful example recently I would mention a group of Universal Sufis from Berlin, who has started in 2013 to recite silent Zikrs and healing prayers on special places who have been wounded by the Nazis or the Stasis.

Let this be a model for us. I am sure, that there are also dark and wounded places in your residence or around it, where you can become active and help to dissolve the evil, to bring light and love and healing with the help of **Allâh.**

Let's do it, inscha **Allâh!**

5

The power of spirit and vibration

The main cause of many physical and mental diseases is the exhaustion of the nerves and thus the weakening of body and mind. And not infrequently imagination does the rest. It makes the person concerned believe to have this or that disease or to fear or to need it. This is precisely where the Sufi teachers and therapists come into play. With a holistic view, they introduce the disciples and clients to an independent control and to self-discipline. Thus, they teach or impart them the importance of the power of the spirit over the body.

The German poet *Novalis* said (200 years ago!): "Every illness is basically a musical problem, the healing is a musical remedy." That's how Sufis see it, too. When the human body loses its originally harmonic state, it becomes ill. Expressed musically: the body rhythm becomes arrhythmic, consonance becomes dissonance, harmony becomes disharmony. Every-thing in both microcosm, and macrocosm is a matter of vibrations. However, health can only be restored and secured if the human being accepts the cosmic unity and its principles and gives himself with all his being. If our mind constantly keeps its thoughts in harmony, it cannot be easily shaken, nervous disorders cannot appear, and physical diseases cannot creep in.

Prayers, meditations and exercises can help us, to rediscover the healthy divine order. The harmony of body and mind of course also depends on other components such as nutrition, way of life, interaction with people, work, and other things.

6

Belief

For a Sufi, the first prerequisite for all healing is the belief in the Lord of the Worlds and His Almighty Work. Treatment and healing solely happens through His Will. Belief is a very intimate and subtle matter, a deeply inner religious and spiritual attitude of the human being. It gives him strength and self-confidence and furthermore possesses a miraculous healing power.

Up until recent times, science smiled at the effects of religious beliefs on body, spirit and soul of humans and dismissed them. But the findings and (healing) successes achieved by belief are sensational. A U.S. study revealed that people who lead a religious life (for example praying in a church, synagogue or mosque) are healthier and have a life expectancy of about 6,6 years longer.

In his book „Timeless healing – the power and biology of belief", the American doctor and scientist *Herbert Benson*, a pioneer in mind body medicine, describes studies and therapies which showed numerous good results such as astonishing assuagements and health improvements in patients. They chose a word, a sentence or a prayer such as „The Lord is my shepherd" or „Be comforted, my soul" and felt more relaxed and healthier in doing so. In his (now) 40 years of work about these phenomenas, *Benson* was able to prove, that religious conviction and belief in one's own recovery or rather a positive attitude have verifiable successes. In his book, *Dr. Benson* writes, that a religious conviction accelerates healing processes. Although the belief in medical recourses is a guarantee for success, experience shows, that the belief in an invincible and omnipotent power is more successful.

In Islam, there are "Six articles of faith". The Muslim or Muslim Sufi believes in:

- the Unity of God, the One God: **Allâh**

- the prophets of God: *Adam, Noah, Abraham, Jacob, Josef, Moses, David, Solomon, Jesus, Muhammad,* and others

- the holy and divinely-revealed books i. e., the Psalter, the Thora (Old Testament), the Bible (New Testament) and the Quran

- the angels: *Gabriel, Michael, Israfil, Azrael,* and others

- the Day of Judgement and the resurrection

- Gods Predestination.

„*There shall be no compulsion in religion*" (Sura al-Baqara, the cow, Sura 2:256), these are my favourite words from the Holy Quran. This means that faith can only be achieved by the grace of **Allâh** and through the free will of man. **God** alone, Who can do everything, is able to guide our hearts.

7

Breath and mindfulness

In the Sufi tradition breath and mindfulness form central themes. Discovering and becoming aware of one's own real breath can cause a change in health and act as an initiation for some searchers. At the very least, it is one of the first impulses on the spiritual path. Observation of breath and special breathing techniques form the basis of each meditation practice. The breath regulates our body in a vital way and is also involved in completely renewing the cells of our body every seven years. In Sufism, special value is also placed on conscious breathing during curative treatments. It leads the practitioner to his real self. Because breath is the secret of life. And it is also the secret of spiritual development, healing, and health.

It is natural to connect the verbal with breathing. After appropriate preparation, the word is taken into the breath and so it becomes a *"Breathing word"*. Inspired by the „Nature meditations" and the associated breathing technique of the great Sufi master *Hazrat Inayat Khan,* I have published a little book in German with the title „Atemworte – Heilworte" („Breathing words – Healing words"). Additionally there is an audio book of the same name, spoken and produced by myself, with accompanying music, which is specially composed for this purpose.

Here is a small selection of the total of 227 meditations for a „mindful living".

Breathing words – healing words (selection)

(Speak the words silently inwardly with inhalation, holding your breath and exhalation, as shown in brackets)

9

I open up (inhale)
„like the flower to the sun" (stop)
to Your Light and Your Love (exhale)

13

His mercy is immeasureable (inhale)
and reaches far beyond earth and heaven (exhale)

134

Wake up from the wrong dream (exhale)
into the real, true being! (inhale)

139

Where is the sense of life? (inhale)
in the absolute being, (exhale)
and the recognition of the self (inhale),
towards the One ... (exhale)

227

... and these breathing and healing words shall have a lasting effect and may come true in His Name, **God** willing, *inscha **Allâh**, âmin!*
(inhale and exhale regularly)

8

The word

The practice of recitation and prayer is an essential element in the life of a Sufi. In the process, the origin holy books are the source for the spiritual remedies and the basis for worship. Words have the power to speak to the cells of the human body. Some especially resonate in the heart, others in the head or in other parts of our body. A Sufi uses certain words as *Mantra* in his recitations (*Zikrs*). These are words or attributes like *Ya Salâm ("O You, Who You are Peace and Salvation")*. During the day, he also always tries to be careful with the choice of words. What could be a better protection against illness and harm than a word or a prayer? The so-called *Basmala* particularly includes vibrant words. All 114 chapters (*Suras)* of the Holy Quran (except the ninth *Sura*) begin with it:

BismiLlâh ir-Rahmân ir-Rahîem

These words could be translated as follows: *In the name of **Allâh**, Most Gracious, Most Merciful.* These words do not only open the daily prayers, but also are spoken before and after certain activities (for example before and after the meals, upon entering and leaving a house, before a drive, etc. They give you energy, courage and protection. Indeed, these words contain every imaginable, infinite blessing.

> *What We are sending down in the course of revealing the Quran is healing and grace for those who have faith.*
> Holy Quran, Sura al-'Isrâ´ (The Journey by Night), Sura 17:82

9

The Beautiful Names of God (al-asmâ' al-husnâ)

> *And to **Allâh** belong the most beautiful names, so invoke Him by them.*
> Holy Quran, Sura Al-A'raf (The Purgatory), Sura 7:180

Meditation respectively recitation of the divine names is balsam for our soul, gives us harmony and healing. *Abu Huraira* narrated: Prophet *Muhammad* – peace and blessings upon him – said, *"**Allâh** has ninety-nine names, i.e. one-hundred minus one, and whoever knows them will go to Paradise"* (Sahih Al-Bukhari, Book 50, Hadith 8949).

ALLÂH The Greatest Name, The Proper Name of God, The One and Only
1 **Ar-Rahmân** The All-Merciful
2 **Ar-Rahîem** The Bestower of Mercy
3 **Al-Malik** The King, The Owner of Dominion
4 **Al-Quddûs** The Holy, The Absolute Pure
5 **As-Salâm** The Peace, The Giver of Peace and Well-Being
6 **Al-Mu'min** The Faithful, The Giver and Guardian of Faith, The Bestower of Security
7 **Al-Muhaymin** The Protector, The Ever-Watchful Guardian
8 **Al-`Aziz** The Almighty, The Strong and Powerful
9 **Al-Jabbâr** The Repairer, The Compeller

10 **Al-Mutakabbir** The Supreme, The Majestic
11 **Al-Khâliq** The Creator, The True Originator
12 **Al-Bâri'** The Evolver, The Maker
13 **Al-Musawwir** The Fashioner, The Shaper
14 **Al-Ghaffâr** The Always and All-Forgiving
15 **Al-Qahhâr** The Subduer, The Dominant
16 **Al-Wahhâb** The Giver of Gifts, The Bestower
17 **Ar-Razzâq** The Provider, The All-Giving
18 **Al-Fattâh** The Opener, The Liberator
19 **Al-`Alîm** The Omniscient, The All-Knowing
20 **Al-Qâbid** The Restrainer, The Constrainer
21 **Al-Bâsit** The Spreader, The Expander
22 **Al-Châfid** The Abaser, The Reducer
23 **Ar-Râfi** The Exalter, The Upraiser
24 **Al-Mu`izz** The Honorer, The Strengthener
25 **Al-Mudhill** The Degrader, The Humiliator
26 **As-Samî`** The All-Hearing
27 **Al-Basîr** The All-Seeing
28 **Al-Hakam** The Judge, The Giver of True Justice
29 **Al-`Adl** The Just, The Equitable
30 **Al-Latîf** The Most Subtle One and Gracious, The Kind
31 **Al-Chabîr** The All-Aware, The Experienced
32 **Al-Halîem** The Most Forbearing, The Clement
33 **Al-`Adhîem** The Magnificent, The Supreme Glory
34 **Al-Ghafûr** The All-Forgiver, The Exceedingly
  Forgiving
35 **Ash-Shakûr** The Most Grateful, The Most Thankful
36 **Al-´Alîy** The Exalted in Might, The Most High
37 **Al-Kabîr** The Most Great, The Unimaginable Great
38 **Al-Hafîz** The Preserver, The Guardian
39 **Al-Muqît** The Sustainer, The Maintainer
40 **Al-Hasîb** The Reckoner, The Calculator
41 **Al-Jalîl** The Sublime One, The Majestic
42 **Al-Karîm** The All Generous, The Noble
43 **Ar-Raqîb** The Watchful, The Observer
44 **Al-Mujîb** The Responsive, The Hearer and Answerer
  Of Prayers
45 **Al-Wâsi** The Comprehensive, The All-Embracing
46 **Al-Hakîm** The Perfectly Wise
47 **Al-Wadûd** The All Loving One
48 **Al-Majîd** The Most Glorious One, The Praiseworthy

49 **Al-Bâ'ith** The Resurrector, The Raiser from Dead
50 **Ash-Shahîd** The Witness of all Things
51 **Al-Haqq** The Absolute Truth, The Reality
52 **Al-Wakîl** The Trustee, The Disposer of all Affairs
53 **Al-Qawî** The Possessor of All Strength
54 **Al-Matîn** The Firm, The Steady
55 **Al-Walîy** The Nearest & Protecting Friend, The Patron
56 **Al-Hamîd** The Only Praiseworthy, The All-Laudable
57 **Al-Muhsî** The Accountant, The Reckoner, The All-Enumerating
58 **Al-Mubdî'** The Originator, The Initiator
59 **Al-Mu`îd** The Restorer, The Reviver of the Dead
60 **Al-Muhyî** The Giver of Life and Health
61 **Al-Mumît** The Bringer of Death, The Destroyer
62 **Al-Hayy** The Alive, The Ever Living and Everlasting
63 **Al-Qayyûm** The Self-Subsisting, The Self-Existing
64 **Al-Wâjid** The Finder, The All-Perceiving
65 **Al-Mâjid** The Noble, The All-Glorious
66 **Al-Wâhid** The One, The Unique One
67 **Al-Ahad** The Only One, The Unity
68 **As-Sâmad** The Eternal-Absolute, The Everlasting
69 **Al-Qâdir** The All Powerful, The Potent and Capable Master
70 **Al-Muqtadir** The Possessor of All Power, The Omnipotent
71 **Al-Muqaddim** The Foremost, The Expediter, The Promoter
72 **Al-Mu'achir** The Delayer, The Retarder
73 **Al-Awwal** The First, The Beginning and The Foremost
74 **Al-Âchir** The Last, The End and The Ultimate
75 **Ad-Dhâhir** The Manifest One, The Evident
76 **Al-Bâtin** The Hidden One, The Internal, The Inmost Secret
77 **Al-Wâli** The Governor, The Friendly and Protecting Ruler
78 **Al-Muta`âli** The Supremely Exalted
79 **Al-Barr** The Righteous, The Source of All Goodness, The All-Benign
80 **At-Tawwâb** The Acceptor of Repentance

81 **Al-Muntaqim** The Avenger
82 **Al-ʿAfûw** The All-Pardoner
83 **Ar-Raʾûf** The Compassionate, The Most Kind
84 **Mâlik-al-Mulk** The Eternal Owner of all Sovereignity, The King of all Kingdoms
85 **Dhûl-Jalâl wal-Ikrâm** The Possessor and Lord of Majesty, Glory and Honour
86 **Al-Muqsit** The Equitable, The Just
87 **Al-Jâmiʾ** The Gatherer, The Assembler of All
88 **Al-Ghanî** The Independent, One, The Rich
89 **Al-Mughnî** The Enricher, The Bestower of Wealth
90 **Al-Mâniʾ** The Preventer, The Withholder
91 **Ad-Dârr** The Distresser, The Afflictor
92 **An-Nâfiʾ** The Benefiter, The Advantageous
93 **An-Nûr** The Light, The Enlightener
94 **Al-Hâdi** The Guide, The Leader
95 **Al-Badîʾ** The Innovative Creator, The Inventor
96 **Al-Bâqi** The Everlasting and Eternal
97 **Al-Wârith** The Supreme Inheritor, The Heir
98 **Ar-Rashîd** The Guide to the Right Path, The Unerring
99 **As-Sabûr** The Most Patient, The Forbearing

During the *Dhikr,* the most beautiful names of **Allâh** are applied as invocations. One example: *Ya Salâm = O You, Who You are Peace* (See also chapter 13 – Zikr, page 50).

10

The Holy Qur'an: Medicine pure

The Holy Quran is a compilation of the verbal revelations given to Prophet *Muhammad* – peace and blessings be upon him - over a period of 23 years. For the Muslims, it lays down the law and commandments, codes for their social and moral behavior and contains a comprehensive religious philosophy. For Muslims the Holy Quran is the book of books. It is full of wonders and blessings. Have you ever asked yourself why so many believers pick up this book again and again, not only in the mosque? The marvellous thing is: The more you read in it, the more you want to read in it. You only read the most books once. But this book never gets boring. It is a powerful work and our language is not capable to express, nor is our human mind able to understand the complete fullness of the Holy Quran. It is divine and inexhaustible. As the saying goes, if the seas were ink, the forests pens, sky and earth paper, and the whole creation would work on a book, it would not be sufficient to explain the meaning of the Holy Quran. It teaches us to be human, it shows us what we must do and what we must not do and how we find the way (back) to **Allâh**, the Guide and the Way. The Holy Quran is the book of God, the book of truth, love and healing. Its words contain every conceivable, indeed eternal blessing.

O mankind! Verily, a warning has come to you from your Lord and a cure for what is in your breasts and guidance and mercy for the believers.
Holy Quran, Sura Yunus (Jonah), Sura 10:57

11

Ritual Prayer

The beneficial and healing effect of the prayer(s) upon creatures has been proved scientifically for a long time. The "Religious Research Foundation", established 1952 in Los Angeles, made studies not only on human beings, but also on plants and animals. It showed that if positive prayers are regularly spoken upon seeds and plants they grow much better.

The postures of *salat*, which are also practiced by the Muslim Sufis, are considered as proto-movements of the angels. They were revealed to the prophet *Muhammad* by the archangel *Jibril (Gabriel)* and have to be performed five times a day. One can indeed compare them with Yoga asanas. There are eight different postures. The effects of this prayer on body, soul, and mind are highly interesting and healing.

The first Sura of the Holy Qur'an, the Sura al-Fâtiha („The Opener"), is recited several times in the aforesaid prayers. It is also called al-Schifâ („The Healing").

The infallible remedy: The Sura al-Fâtiha

The Prophet – peace be upon him – said: "In Sura al-Fâtiha there is a balm for all ailments." He went on to provide the specific instructions for utilizing this most treasured remedy. He also said: "I tell you of a surah that is the greatest, the most virtuous, in the Holy Qur'an. It is Sura al-Hamd (the opening Sura, al-Fâtiha), which has seven

---

verses. These are the sab'ah mathani (the Oft-Repeated Seven) and represent the Grand Qur'an."

In another hadith, the Prophet – peace and blessings be upon him – is reported to have said: "By Him Who is in possession of my life, a sura like this one has been revealed neither in the Tora, nor in the Bible, nor even in the rest of the Qur'an."

The accumulated experience of the Sufis confirms that the reading and reciting of Sura al-Fâtiha with true faith and sincere conviction, cures all maladies, whether spiritual or worldly, external or internal. The Sura al-Fâtiha enters into the writing of almost all ta'widh; it is also written in ink made of saffron and rose water, and consumed. All six books of authentic (sahih) Hadith report that the companions – may **Allâh** be pleased with them - used to read it for treatment of diseases, both physical and mental.

The satan lamented, wept, and tore his hair out on four occasions; when he was cursed, when he was thrown out of Heaven, when Muhammad – peace and blessings be upon him – was given prophethood, and when Sura al-Fâtiha was revealed.

Hazrat Khwaja Moinuddin Chishti – may **Allâhs** blessing be with him - has said: "The incessant recitation of Sura al-Fâtiha is the infallible remedy for one's needs."

The recitation of Sura al-Fâtiha is among the most frequent of the practices of the shaykhs of the path. The Prophet Muhammad – peace and blessings be upon him – suggested the following mode of recitation and said that this practice will succeed in curing any disease:

Read Sura al-Fâtiha forty-one times for forty consecutive days, during the interval between

the *sunna (optional)* and *fard (obligatory) ra'kats* of the fair (early-morning) prayer. In this recitation, it is necessary to omit the breath pause usually taken between the first two verses. In other words, the *mim* of ir-Rahîm is joined with the *lam* of *al-hamdu li-Llâhi,* which then becomes *mil-hamdu li-Llâhi. The rest of the Sura may be done following the usual breath pauses.*

If the person is possessed of madness, or for other reasons cannot perform the recitation, the words should be recited and blown on water, and given to the patient to drink.

Source: www.chishti.org

Here are the lyrics of the Sura al-Fatiha in Arabic, in Arabic pronunciation or transliteration and analogous English translation:

بِسْمِ اللهِ الرَّحْمٰنِ الرَّحِيمِ

الْحَمْدُ لِلّهِ رَبِّ الْعَالَمِينَ الرَّحْمٰنِ الرَّحِيمِ

مَالِكِ يَوْمِ الدِّينِ إِيَّاكَ نَعْبُدُ وَإِيَّاكَ

نَسْتَعِينُ اهْدِنَا الصِّرَاطَ الْمُسْتَقِيمَ

صِرَاطَ الَّذِينَ أَنْعَمْتَ عَلَيْهِمْ

غَيْرِ الْمَغْضُوبِ عَلَيْهِمْ وَلَا الضَّالِّينَ

BismilLâh ir-rahmân ir-rahîm
al-hamdu li-llâhi rabbi-l-'alamîn
ar-rahmân ir-rahîm
maliki yaum-id-dîn
iyyâka na'budu wa iyyâka nasta'în
ihdinâs-sirât al-mustaqîm
sirât alladhîna an'amta 'alayhim
ghayril-maghdûbi 'alayhim wa lâd-dâlin

*In the name of **Allâh**, Most Gracious, Most Merciful,*
*All praises and thanks be to **Allâh**, the Lord of the Universe,*
Most Gracious, Most Merciful,
Master of the day of judgement.
You Alone we worship, and You Alone we ask for Help.
Guide us the straight way,
The Way of those whom You have favored; not of Those who have earned Your wrath, or of those Who have lost the way.

The postures of the Muslim prayer

The ritual Muslim prayer is performed with following postures:

• **Standing up straight** improves body posture, deepens concentration and trains awareness.

• **Bending** strengthens muscles and bones and leads to inner harmony.

• **Prostration** stimulates the muscles and the circulation, it is also very beneficial for pregnant women. It is a posture of patience, humility, and trust in God.

- **The sitting posture** is helpful for stomach, intestine, liver, and a good digestion.

Depending on the time of day or night the respective prayers are spoken loudly or internally. Through the vibrations of the long vowels, heart, thyroid gland, pineal gland, pituitary gland, lungs and kidneys are stimulated and purified. If one respects the prayer times, he is in complete tune with the movements of the planets, the change of seasons, and the geographical differences, therefore in harmony with the natural cyclic courses in the universe.

The meals of the Sufis are also introduced, accompanied and terminated by prayers. They have a harmonizing, beneficial and healing effect on the diner.

Nazar* - Grace

O Thou, the Sustainer
Of our bodies, hearts and souls,
Bless all that we receive in thankfulness.
Amen.

Hazrat Inayat Khan

Nayaz** - Healing prayer

Beloved Lord, Almighty God!
Through the rays of the sun,
Through the waves of the air,
Through the all-pervading life in space,
Purify and revivify me, and, I pray,
Heal my body, heart and soul.
Amen.

Hazrat Inayat Khan

* = sacrifice; ** = deference

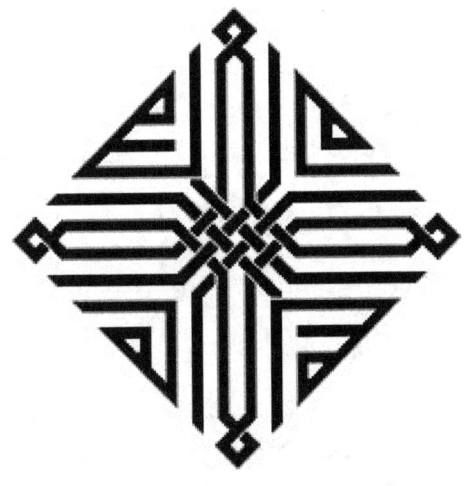

„La ilaha illa **LIâh**"

12

The Keys to the Treasures of Heaven and Earth *(Maqualad as-samawati wal ard)*

In principle you should recite the following two verses before every Sufi exercise for protection from negative influences:

Lâ ilâha illâ **Llâh**, *Muhammadan rasûlu* **Llâh**.
(There is no God but **Allâh** and *Muhammad* is His messenger)

and

*A`udhu bi-***Llâh***i mina sch-schaytân ir-radschîem.*
(I seek **Allâhs** protection from Satan, the rejected one).

One of the central chapters in the marvelous work THE BOOK OF SUFI HEALING of *Sheikh Hakim abu Abdullah Moinuddin al Chishtiyya* is „The Treasures of Heavens and Earth", in Arabic: *„Maqualad as-samawati wal ard".* They belong to the most powerful healing words of all.

Lâ ilâha illâ **Llâh***u wa-***Llâh***u akbar*
wa subhân **Allâh***u wal-hamdu li-***Llâh***i*
wastaghfiru **Llâh** *alladhî lâ ilâha illâ Hû*
wa-Awwalu wal-Âkhiru waz-Zâhiru wal-Bâtinu
yuhyi wa yumîtu wa huwa Hayyan lâ yamûtu
bi-yadihil-khayr wa huwa `alâ kulli schay´in Qadîr.

> *There is none worthy of worship except **Allâh**,*
> ***Allâh** is the greatest,*
> ***Allâh** is the glorious and praiseworthy*
> *and I ask **Allâh** for forgiveness.*
> *There is no power to do good*
> *and no strength to be saved from evil*
> *except with the grace of **Allâh**.*
> *He is the First and the Last,*
> *He is the Apparent and the Hidden,*
> *in His hand lies all good,*
> *He is the Giver of life and death,*
> *He has ability over everything.*

As a reward for the recitation of this verse, the original text of the said book reads: The Prophet – peace and blessing be upon Him – continues (in a conversation with `Uthmân Ibn `Affân – may **Allâh** be pleased with him): „O `Uthmân, anyone who recites that one hundred times every day will be rewarded with ten graces:

Firstly, all his past sins will be forgiven.

Secondly, he is released from suffering from the fires of hell.

Thirdly, two angels will be assigned to protect him day and night against suffering and illness.

Fourthly, he will receive a treasure of blessing.

Fifthly, he will harvest as much blessing as somebody who releases 100 slaves from the tribe of the Prophet *Ismael* – peace upon Him.

Sixthly, he will be rewarded with the blessing that he would receive if he would read the whole Qur'an, the Psalms, the Tora, and the Bible.

43

Seventhly, a house is built for him in heaven.

Eighthly, he will be married to a pious heavenly woman.

Ninthly, he will be crowned with a crown of honor,

and tenthly, his recommendations (for forgiveness) concerning seventy of his relatives will be accepted.

O `Uthmân, if you were strong enough, you would not miss a single day of this remembrance. You will belong to the successful persons and surpass anyone who was before you or comes after you."

13

Zikr

> Truly, in rememberance of **Allâh** hearts become peaceful.
> Holy Qur'an, Sura Ar-Ra'd (The thunder), Sura 13:28

> O you who have believed, remember **Allâh** with much remembrance. And exalt Him in the morning and in the evening.
> Holy Qur'an, Sura Al-Ahzab (The Combined Forces), Sura 33:41-42

Zikr or *Zikru**Llâh*** (also *Zekr, Dhikr, Sikr*) means „rememberance". This rememberance goes back to the very first dialogue with **God**, the Almighty. The original question He once asked His creatures was: „*Alastu bi-Rabbikum?*" = „*Am I not Your Lord?*" It is written in the Holy Quran, Sura Al-A'raaf (The Heights), Sura 7:172. They said: „*Yes indeed! We bear witness.*" Human beings have forgotten this „covenant of love", as it is called. But in deep prayer and meditation and ecstatic dance we can hear the divine call : „*Alastu bi-Rabbikum?*". Mevlana Rumi, the great Sufi master and poet says: „*Anyone who only has a dream of the Alastu day, will be intoxicated on the way full of devotion.*"

During a *Zikr* holy verses, the *Shahada* or Holy Names of **God** are recited or sung. *Zikr* is the huge source of strength for the practitioners. It is possible to practice it alone or in a group, which sometimes can be big. The *Zikr* may slightly differ in the form and the procedure from order to order.

Among traditional dervishes, it is said that a *Zikr* of less than four hours would be nothing but a waste of time. The Sufi mystic *Ibn Arabi* (1165-1240) considers the name of God „**Allâh**" as the most valuable means for continual remembrance.

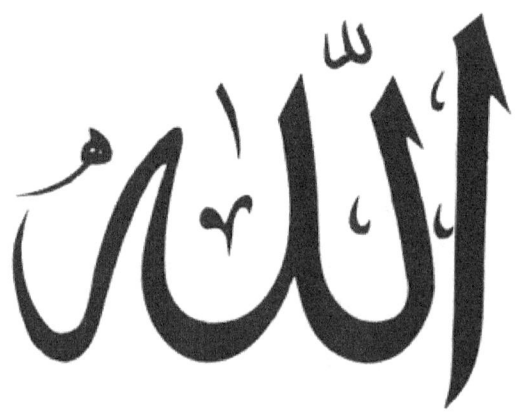

Meditation and Zikr exercise „Allâh"

Copy the above Arabic word „**Allâh**" (best of all, in an enlarged form). Take this as a basis for your meditation. Place the sheet of paper in front of you and begin by looking at it calmly. Meditate on the forms of the word. The name **Allâh** represents a path:

ALIF
LAM
LAM
HA

The first letter of the Arabian alphabet ALIF also symbolizes the beginning of life. The two LAM letters represent the path, the duality. And the HA may symbolize the end, death, but at the same time resurrection and birth. This letter also represents the transition of the subject feeling from the self to God. *Ibn Arabi* comments: *„The letter HA symbolizes something that is absent. It represents the condition of the non-manifestation of the pure essence."* In this calligraphy, feminine and masculine attributes can also be discovered. Now speak following the rhythm **„Al-lâh, Al-lâh, Al-lâh, Al-lâh ..."**, breath after every fourth **Allâh**.

The classical Zikr

In the following, you can see the procedure of a classical *Zikr* as it is practiced in many orders:

Lâ ilâha îlla Llâh (Hu)

Prior to the ritual, a preparation, attunement or cleaning (in Muslim orders *Wudû')* shall take place.

Here, the classical *Zikr* is carried out sitting using the words *„Lâ ilâha îlla* **Llâh**" and is connected with a dynamic movement.

At the beginning („Lâ"), the head is tilted slightly downwards to the left towards the heart. Then, it makes a circular movement from bottom to top („ilâha"), past the right shoulder, then falls slightly backwards and moves back down towards the heart over the left shoulder („îlla") and remains there for some time („Llâh"). In some ordes, a „Hu" is also added.

The Tesbih

For the recitation of the Zikr, you should use a *Tesbih*. It is helpful while reciting *Wazifas*, the beautiful names of **God**, and other *Zikr* formulas. It is assumed that the Sufis and Muslims „copied" them from the *Mala* of the Buddhists. The *Tesbih* consists mostly of wooden beads, but may also be made of seed balls, olive stones, pearls, glass, or plastic. It has 33, 99 or 100 beads; necklaces with 11 or 1000 are also common. In the early Islamic time, believers recited the beautiful names of **God** by means of small stones or with their fingers. Strictly orthodox Muslims like the Wahhabis reject a *Tesbih* as an innovation (*bid'a*). However, the friend of the Prophet *Muhammad* – peace and blessings be upon him -, the first Caliph *Abu Bakr*, is supposed to have already used one. Hold the *Tesbih* with the left and right hand and count the individual beads or rather move them with the forefinger of the right hand. If you are sitting on the floor, you should never let the *Tesbih* touch the floor. I personally always carry a *Tesbih* with me, in the pocket of my trousers or jacket or worn around the hand or neck. Apart from my silver wedding ring, it is the only thing that I carry with me 24 hours. It has become a basic need for me to practice the everlasting *Zikr* with it.

Walking Zikr

I gained the first practical experiences with the *Walking Zikr* at the lectures in the *international Sufi summer school* in Katwijk aan Zee (Holland). And then in the following winter in the snowy landscape of a Hessian village idyll. In the Sufi group at that time, we practiced the *Zikr „Ischq **Allâh** mahbûd* *li*/**Lâh**". These were amazing adventures and experiences. Here we recited this *Zikr* loudly and made one step with every syllable. After some time, we spoke softer and softer and took the words into the breath. The *Walking Dhikr* has an intensively cleaning, clarifying, God uniting effect.

The Hadra

The Arabic word *Hadra* means present, presence (of **God**). The gathering of the Dervishes and Sufis, which traditionally takes place after sunset and where *Zikr* and ecstatic dances or rather movements are performed, is also referred to as *Hadra*. The Dervish group repeats the beautiful names of **God** and a soloist, usually the Sheikh of the order, sings hymn-like melodies about them. The ceremonial highlight is often the intensive exclaiming of the words „**Allâh**" and „**Hu**", accompanied by the participants breathing out and in deeply. As they breathe out, they bend forward, as they breathe in, they rise up again with a slight movement backwards. In some orders, the Sheikh also gives a short lecture as part of the event, answers questions and provides information about internal matters and various events. Afterwards there is a common meal with a final prayer or rather invocation.

Significant Zikrs and Wazifas

Allâh (= Allâh, **God**)
See figure and exercise page 46

Hu (= He is)
This name has even deeper, mystical meanings and is considered the most perfect among the names of God.

AllâHu* (= God is)

Lâ illâha îlla Llâh* (= There is no god but **God**)

33times **Subhâna-Llâh** (=Glory be to **Allâh**)

33times **Al-hâmduli-Llâh** (= Praise be to **Allâh**)

33times **Allâhu akbar** (= **Allâh** is bigger than anything we could imagine)

AstârchfiruLlâh* (= **God**, forgive us)
A tremendous *Zikr* which allows the great power of forgiveness to develop and can make enemies become friends.

Bismi Llâh ir-Rahmân ir-Rahîem (= In the name of **God**, the Gracious, the Merciful)
This formula is referred to as *Basmala*. A special blessing originates from it. It can not only be recited as *Zikr*, but also during the entire everyday life as a protection and blessing formula (e. g., before meals, when leaving the house, before trips and journeys, etc.).

Ya Hayyû, ya Qayyûm (= o You, who is alive, o You, who lasts forever!)
According to some Sufis, these two attributes together form the greatest name of **Allâh**.

Lâ illâha îlla LIâh, ya Allâh, ya Haqq, ya Hayy, ya Hu, ya Qayyûm, ya Qahhâr*
(= There is no god but **God**, o **Allâh**, o You, who is the truth, o You, who is alive, o You, who you are, o You, who lasts forever, o You invincible)
This *Zikr* originates from the tradition of the *Qadiriyya* Sufis.

Ya Latîfu, ya Kâfi, ya Hafîdhu, ya Schâfi, ya Karimu, ya Baqi, ya Rahimu, ya Allah* (= o Friendly, o Allmighty, o Guardian, o Healer, o Noble, o Endurer, o Merciful, o **God**)
This *healing Zikr* was taught to me by *Efendi Mehmet Ungan*, singer and Ud player of the music group *Hosh Neva* and leader of the oriental music school in Mannheim (Germany). He composed a melody for it which can be heard on the CD *Mantras heal the World*.

Subhân Allâh wa bihâmdihi
(= Blessed be **Allâh** und thanks to Him)
According to a Hadith, these are the words which are most loved by **Allâh**.

La hâula wa la qûwatta îlla bîLlah
(= There is no power and no strength except for **Allâh**)
This formula, called *Hauqala,* offers a special protection against *Djinns* and negative people. Additionally, it gives rest, peace, and healing. In a *Hadith* it states that it is a remedy against 90 diseases. It is also helpful in cases of sorrow and depression.

*You can find musical notes of these zikrs or wazifas in my SUFI SONGBOOK (sol music). See also page 90.

14

Meditation

In meditation, there are unsuspected powers and boundless blessing.
Yan d'Albert

Meditation is a „24-hour job" for the Sufi, he actually sees his whole life as one single meditation. Even scientists were able to prove that meditation strengthens the immune system, the heart, and the circulation and reduces anxiety states. Meditation helps in cases of stress, fear, high blood pressure, or also pain. Mental states and physical well-being are undoubtedly closely connected. The regular practice of meditating does not only change your thinking and feeling in a positive way, your whole life takes a completely new turn. You develop a deeper understanding of the meaning of existence. Finally, your insights shine on your own life and on that of others. This allows you to permanently find more harmony, happiness, and health. This is the real meaning of meditation.

Meditation practice:

1 Go into yourself and immerse yourself in silence.
2 Open up to the light and to the inspiration.
3 Practice concentration (e. g. on words).
4 Control your breath.
5 Observe yourself closely.
6 Find the source of your real power.
7 Trace which insight you gain from meditation.

(translated from: „Atemworte – Heilworte, Geführte Meditationen für ein achtsames Leben", Yan d'Albert, edition sol 2016.)

15

Salvific virtues

I tried to call attention to virtues in my book „The 66 virtues of the Sufis" (Latest title: „The book of the 66 virtues"). Many of them are increasingly being forgotten.

Here are some of them:

FORGIVENESS

Forgiveness brings solution.
Solution leads to salvation.
And salvation means healing.
Yan d'Albert

Don't waste any time, but rather forgive a person immediately. Accept his apology straight away. Both you and the respective person will develop blockades due to non-forgiving. As a result, you will form real knots in your body and thus, your stream of life can no longer flow freely. How else can all these illnesses be explained?: stomach ulcers, headaches, cramps, paralyses, and more. There are indeed means and possibilities to dissolve these blockades, by forgiving without compromise, by saying prayers, by meditating and also expressing this in a singing manner. But remember: actually, only **God** can really forgive, and He does this gladly and all the time.

Meditation of forgiving

Close your eyes, relax, breath calmly and regularly. Then think of a person you currently have problems with, but you care deeply about a quick solution. Imagine the following like a movie: let this person walk back and forth before your eyes. Visualize how annoyed he is, how he shouts, how nasty and aggressive he is towards you, and how he deeply hurts you. After a short break, think of his positive characteristics. Maybe this person is hiding a soft core behind a hard shell. Maybe he has virtues like punctuality and reliability. Now try to find something positive on the person's body. Maybe he has beautiful hands that can tackle things in a helpful and reliable manner. Now send light to this spot and let it become stronger from there and spread on the entire body. When the person is completely wrapped in light, speak words of forgiveness with a smile, give the smile to him!

PURITY

A clean body reflects the purity of the soul and is the secret of health.
Hazrat Inayat Khan

The purpose of ritual purity and washings in the different traditions and religions (e. g. in Islam, in Hinduism, and others) is to purify body, mind, and soul, to prepare for meditation and prayer, to open up to the Deity or to **God**. For the Muslim, or rather the Muslim Sufi, purity is a duty. The ritual washing before prayers is called *wudû´*. The five daily prayers *(sâlat)* are only allowed to be performed in a state of internal and external physical purity and in a clean place. The prayer has no effect without purity.

But purity does not only include the physical purity, this also widely means moral, virtuous characteristics: purity of thoughts, attitude, and actions.

The purity of a spiritual person also includes environmental protection. Therefore, I did not shy

55

away from calling awareness of environmental protection a virtue, too.

ENVIRONMENTAL AWARENESS

> *Today's humanity consequently behaves as if they were driven by the devil who has the sole target to destroy all life on our planet.*
> Konrad Lorenz

Anyone who wants to live healthy, should consequently also behave in an environmentally aware manner.

The planet on which we live, called earth, is God's creation. Very clearly. It is **God's** gift to us. We are not able to create a single seed, a leaf on the tree, lakes and oceans, neither wind nor rain or snow, neither thunder nor lightning.

Everybody has the opportunity to contribute something towards protecting the nature and environment, for example:

•   To be economical in the use of our precious water,

•   to avoid buying plastic products,

•   to only undertake really necessary car trips,

•   to generally limit the personal consumption,

•   and a lot more ...

Live environmentally aware every day!

HEALTH AWARENESS

> *Eat and drink from what **Allâh** prepared for you and do not cause disaster on earth!*
> Holy Quran, Sura al-Baqara (the cow), Sura 2:60

This Quran sentence expresses a highly topical demand. What should we eat? We should eat what **Allâh**, the All-Sublime, prepared for us. And this clearly means natural food and not artificially produced products such as extruder food or fast food.

The attributes or virtues of a person who lives a consciously spiritual or religious life include health awareness. With the attitude towards health, we have a great responsibility for ourselves and our children, towards our fellow human beings and future generations.

Here, too, as in the case with many other questions of life, the Sufi uses his common sense and relies upon the divine inspiration and guidance of his Creator.

Eat health-consciously every day!

16

Sayings of the Prophet
peace and blessings be upon Him –

(selection)

Less food, less sin.

The stomach is the home of disease and abstinence the head of every remedy. So make this your custom.

There is blessing in three things: in the early morning meal, in bread and in soup.

Allow your food to cool before eating, for in hot food there is no blessing.

Eat together and then disperse, for a blessing resides in groups.

In the sight of **Allâh**, the best food is a food shared by many.

Use *miswak*, for this practice comes from cleanliness, and cleanliness comes from faith, and faith takes its practitioner to heaven.

Allâh said that he who lives according to the Qur'an will have a long live.

*"O **Allâh** cure my body, cure my heart and cure my eyesight from any illness."* (repeated 3 times)

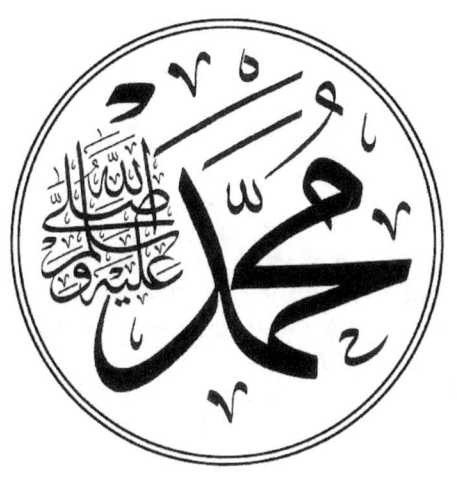

"Muhammad -
peace and blessings be upon Him"

17

Preferred healing food and application

Sufis pay attention to the choice of their food products and thus to good nutrition. The conscious preparation, accompanied by prayers and chants, is just as important for them.

When the Prophet *Muhammad* – peace and blessings upon Him – was once asked why he and his companions enjoyed such excellent health, he answered: *„We always eat together, and we are moderate. And we only eat when we are hungry and we prefer to leave something before we eat a bite too much."*

For many Sufis, the doctrine of the four essences of the human body (arab.: *akhlât*) according to the Persian doctor *Avicenna* (980-1037) serves as basis for nutrition. These are:

blood essence: hot and humid
phlegm essence: cold and humid
gall essence: hot and dry
melancholy essence: cold and dry

The characteristics cold, humid, hot, and dry, or combinations thereof are assigned to food (e. g. butter = hot, humid; salt = hot, dry, etc.). The four essences of the physical body are involved in the digestive process and take effect in the liver. From there, the valuable nutrients enter the bloodstream via the heart as a blood essence. When digesting the remaining nutrients, the less valuable amount becomes a phlegm essence and is converted into mucus, saliva, and gastric juice. The other substances become a gall essence which has an effect on the small intestine and the blood. Finally, the residues are converted into the melancholy essence which passes into the blood and spleen and mixes with the phlegm essence. The aim of the treatment is to achieve a natural balance of the essences.

Our food situation

Our food situation across the world has changed dramatically. We should not simply eat what we are being offered without any concern, especially by the food industry whose products, quite frankly, poison us more and more. If we want to live healthy, we cannot avoid to critically examine these and to constantly inform ourselves.

We have exploited, exhausted, and contaminated our soils, destroyed masses of forests, fished-out and polluted the seas. Accordingly, our food has become contaminated. In my research thereon (particularly about cancer-causing food products) for a new book project, I was increasingly shocked by the many disease-causing ingredients.

It appears that we cannot manage without particular, selected, and nutrient-rich food and food supplement in the future.

In the following, I have made a list of food products which Sufis preferably eat. These also include some special ones, I call them „wonder food": e. g. *argan oil, spirulina, chlorella, moringa,* and more.

List of preferred healing food:

ALGAE have phenomenal effects. The world of algae is full of fascination and hides unimaginable wealth. It is estimated that 200.000 types exist, of which about 40.000 are known. Algae and their ingredients are used for a wide range of purposes, including the food production (vegetables, salad, etc.), food supplement, energy production, and more. Science and medicine are constantly occupied with investigating the health effects of algae, particularly with developing new antibiotics and anti-cancer agents from them. After all, for example, more than 70 substances that attack and destroy cancer cells effectively have been discovered in algae so far. Thereby, especially brown and red algae give rise to great hope. So, ecology scientists certified that they have a whole arsenal of previously unknown molecules that could fight diseases like cancer, HIV, and hepatitis. Algae, which are opposed to strong sunlight in the sea, inhibit the respective viruses far more effectively. Spirulina, chlorella, and AFA algae belong to the most well-known and previously most effective algae types from which products like powder, capsules, tablets, and bath additives are made.

APPLES strengthen the heart and harmonize the body. They have a blood-purifying effect and stimulate the metabolism. Additionally, apples are effective against diarrhea and constipation, vitamin deficiency, and gout. There is an English saying: „An apple a day keeps the doctor away".

ARGAN, the „liquid gold of the desert", is a universal miracle cure against all kinds of diseases. The dear God meant it well with the South Moroccans, because the argan trees only grow in the area of the southern Atlas Mountains: the goats in this area are so wild about the argan nuts that they specially climb the trees to pick them. The Berber women produce the precious healing oil through laborious handcraft. They use it internally and externally, as finest oil in the kitchen, and as care product and remedy for skin and hair. Further application areas in naturopathy include, for example, neurodermitis, acne, eczema, reduction of the cancer risk, joint diseases, cardiovascular problems, dyslipidemia, Alzheimer's and Parkinson's diseases.

BLACK CUMIN OIL is a true miracle remedy. The Sufis say that it heals every disease except for death. It is produced from the seeds of real black cumin. In the Orient, it has been used as medicine for more than 2000 years. Amongst other things, it helps in the case of asthma, with chemotherapies for the mitigation of side effects, with cardiovascular diseases, indigestion, pregnancy-related problems, skin care, and diets.

The Sufi prefers to bake **BREAD** himself, made of the finest whole grain flour. As he gives due honor to it, he does not like to cut the bread with a knife, but rather breaks it with his hands.

COFFEE is actually an invention of the Sufis. Until today, it is a traditional favorite drink which also accompanies them through the long nights of meditation, praying, and dancing. It is stated that coffee (in moderate doses) inspires, strengthens the heart, and evokes wisdom. According to recent studies, the regular consumption of coffee is also supposed to be a very effective remedy against cancer.

DATES are so nourishing that seven of them would be enough food to get through a day (an ideal desert provision!). Traditionally on fasting days or rather during Ramadan, the fasting is broken with a date.

The **FIG** is called the fruit of paradise and is mentioned as nourishing food in many books (also in the Holy Quran in Sura At-Tîn (the fig). It is recommended, e. g., for gout, hemorrhoids, rheumatism, and constipation.

GARLIC is a must in every meal of the Sufis. Due to its antibacterial, disinfecting, antispasmodic, and cancer-preventing effect, it is a good remedy against arteriosclerosis, thus prevents heart attacks and strokes, helps in cases of infections, loss of appetite, and indigestion. Garlic cleans the body and strengthens the immune system. According to recent studies, it is supposed to kill 13 types of infections and 14 types of cancer.

GINGER, or rather the ginger root, is a tropical and subtropical plant whose underground part, the tuber, is used in the kitchen and in medicine. Ginger has an enormous anti-inflammatory and analgesic effect (antioxidants). The spicy substances are similar to the active ingredient in aspirin, acetyl salicin acid. For example, by taking ginger extract in cases of joint inflammations, a significant improvement and pain relief is achieved. Ginger keeps the blood fluid and thus the cells healthy. Externally, ginger can also be used to decrease irritation in the case of wounds. Internally, it also helps in cases of travel sickness (vomiting), indigestion, and loss of appetite. It should be ensured that ginger is not dosed too high because that could cause stomach and intestinal cramps in sensitive persons. Researchers from the *Georgia State University* have found out that ginger was able to reduce the size of a prostate tumor in mice up to 56%.

HENNA is a universal remedy and is recommended for many disease states: it has a germ-killing effect and is used for skin diseases. It is also supposed to be a good remedy against the „evil eye". Henna is ideally suited as natural and healthy hair dye. In the Orient, women traditionally use it at weddings and festivities for coloring their hands and feet. By the way, the perfume produced from henna blossoms is considered as one of the best in the world. And the scent is known for activating the passions of love.

HONEY is regarded as *the* ultimate food product and remedy among the Sufis. The Prophet Muhammad said: *„When somebody eats honey, a thousand remedies enter his stomach and one million diseases leave him"*. He himself used to drink a glass of honey water every morning on an empty stomach.

LENTILS were praised by seventy (!) prophets and recommended by the Sufis as a remedy against cancer diseases. They are one of the oldest crops and were already cultivated in Egypt and Asia Minor 10.000 years ago. There are dozens of kinds in different colors and shapes around the world. Lentils are rich in B-vitamins, fiber, and minerals: calcium, potassium, magnesium, copper, phosphorus, zinc, and especially large amounts of iron.

MORINGA, with the full botanical name *„Moringa oleifera"*, comes from the Himalaya. It is a true miracle tree and is also referred to as „tree of long life". In Ayurveda, the healing power has been known for centuries. When reading the unbelievably long list and the many effects, you can really get dizzy. Nearly all nutrients that we need for our health are available in blossoms, leaves, fruits, bark, roots, and seeds: plenty of protein, numerous minerals (magnesium, calcium, potassium, iron), vitamins (A, B1, B2, C, E), 18 amino acids, 26 substances with an anti-inflammatory effect, and 46 antioxidative substances. More than 700 studies prove the health-promoting and even very cancer-inhibiting effect of this panacea.

The **OLIVE** provides a very healing oil. Here in the West, the numerous healing effects are only really being discovered in recent times. It is used for the treatment of the skin, for eczema, neurodermitis, externally and internally in case of colds. It strengthens the liver, helps in cases of constipation and high blood pressure. The olive oil, e. g. from Morocco, has a particularly good quality and effect.

PEPPERMINT is drunk as tea or used as essential oil. Internally, it is used in cases of indigestion and stomach cramps, externally in cases of colds and sinusitis.

The **POMEGRANATE** is a true miracle fruit. It is mentioned several times in the Old Testament of the Bible and also in the Holy Quran in Sura Al-An´am (the cattle). The fruit is very nutritious, rich in calcium, sodium, niacin, phosphorus, riboflavin, and thiamine. According to *Hadith,* pomegranate cleans the stomach and the seeds should also be eaten.

SAFFRON originates from the Orient. Researchers were able to prove an antioxidant, cancer-inhibiting effect in saffron. In high doses, it can show toxic effects and should therefore not be used as a medicine.

According to a Hadith (= statement of the Prophet *Muhammad*), **SALT** heals more than seventy illnesses. Traditionally, the Sufis eat a pinch of salt before each meal. For this purpose, a few grains are picked up with moistened fingertips and placed on the tongue. The salt stimulates the gastric and digestive juices and the appetite.

The **ONION** is essential in the kitchen and in nature medicine. For the Sufis, raw pressed onion juice is one of the cures for cancer: as a therapy, half a Turkish tea glass of onion juice should be drunk first thing every morning on an empty stomach for 40 days.

VINEGAR was used by all prophets. Mixed with rose water, an excellent healing remedy against toothache and headache is created. An excellent fasting cure and detox treatment can be made with vinegar, at best with organic, pure cider vinegar. The excretory organs such as skin, lung, intestine, and kidney are activated, and toxic waste products and slags are excreted. Additionally, cider vinegar prevents potassium and mineral deficiency during the cure.

18

„Attar" – the magical oil and the „maqams" – the states of the soul

The oil, which is made from a blossom, a wood, or a bark, is called *Attar*. The Sufis do not only see it as oil or essence, but also as the soul of the plant. *Attars* are used at gatherings, common prayers, celebrations, and for healing. The Sufis assign certain m*aqams*, states of the soul, to the *attars*, or rather use them for these. For example, there are states of egoism, heart, soul, the divine secrets, closeness, and union with the divine. As can be indicated by the order, these are spiritually progressive states which can be experienced during the training of the Sufi. There are several possibilities to use the oils physically. Traditionally, the disciple receives the oil with the outstretched right hand, with the palm facing downwards, from the *Sheikh* or teacher. Then he rubs it onto his chin and his wrists and strokes over his clothes. Particularly for the treatment of emotional or mental states, a few drops of oil are applied to the right outer ear. In the Chinese acupuncture, the spot on the ear where this is applied is known as *shen wen,* an important energetic spot. Here are the most widely used *Attars* of the Sufis:

AMBER (*Pers.:* kahrabah) is produced from the pine species *Picea succinfera*. Amber helps in cases of disorders and diseases of the heart. It is particularly effective to apply one drop of it to the „third eye". That stimulates the pineal gland which in turn activates many physiological functions. The best amber types come from the Near East, Russia, and der Dominican Republic.

DSCHANNAT AL-FARDAUS *(Arab.)* means something like „gateway to the highest heaven". It is supposed to once have been composed by a Sufi scent creator when he got to the highest heaven during his mystical practices. After he returned, he tried to produce the scent he perceived there. Dschannat al-Fardaus is used in Sufi medicine.

The oil produced from the blossoms of the henna plant (see effects!) is called **HINA**. It is one of the finest and most valuable oils in the world. It can be stored for a long period of time, whereby its quality is improved.

INCENSE is a very effectively cleaning meditation and ritual oil. Since it, depending on the variety, can have a very intensive effect, it should be used with particular caution. It purifies both the atmosphere and the human aura of negative vibrations.

JASMINE has a pain-relieving effect as a compress, and an aphrodisiac, relaxing, and harmonizing effect as body or bath oil. It helps in cases of depression, lifts the spirits, and strengthens the self-confidence.

The Prophet *Muhammad* – peace and blessing upon Him – described **MUSK** as having the most pleasant odor. It is produced from the gonads of an antelope species. Musk is used in cases of inner unrest and dysphoria, clears the thoughts, and warms up the limbs. It also heals the heart and has an aphrodisiac effect.

MYRRH is a component of holy anointing oils. *Moses* (or *Musa*) and *Jesus* (or *Eisa*) – peace upon them – already received it as a gift from God. Myrrh was already used in the early days for cleaning and purification, for dedications and rituals. It is anti-inflammatory, balancing, meditation-supporting, and perfect for cleaning the room air.

ROSE – depending on the type (there are about 300 different types of roses worldwide!), it has different characteristics. Real rose oil is very expensive. The Bulgarian, Indian, and Moroccan oils are particularly fine. Rose is calming, spirits-lifting, and heart-opening. Rose oil is also used for skin care and as an eye bath in cases of eye inflammations.

SANDALWOOD is also a ritual oil, perfect for meditations and mental practices. It has a woody, exotic scent and has a warming, sensual, and inspiring effect. Sandalwood improves its quality with increasing age.

TEA TREE OIL is a true miracle cure. It cleans, stimulates, and strengthens, and fights bacteria, viruses, and fungi quickly and successfully.

'UD is the oil produced from the Aloe tree. It is used in cases of mental imbalances.

The *Attars* can be assigned to the respective states of the soul or be used for these:

Maqam an-nafs (state of egotism): jasmine, musk, rose, sandalwood, incense (physical); - rose, violet, incense (mental)

Maqam al-qalb (state of the heart): amber, musk, rose (physical); - jasmine, sandalwood, violet, incense (mental)

Maqam ar-ruh (state of the soul): amber, hina, musk, 'ud (physical); - rose, sandalwood, violet (mental)

Maqâm as-sirr (state of the divine secrets): Dschannat al-Fardaus (physical); - hina, sandalwood, 'ud, (mental)

Maqâm al-qurb (state of closeness): amber, rose (mental)

Maqâm al-wisal (state of the divine union): rose

Arabic aromatic oils or *Attars* which are mixed with various other oils are also commercially available.

19

The *Ta`wîdh* - formula and amulet of salvific symbols

Similar to the classical magic, the Sufis use certain formulas and amulets for healing purposes, too.

A *Ta`wîdh* is a formula or amulet which contains verses from the Holy Quran (and is allowed in Islam), similarly, often also numbers. The principle is based on the number symbolism of the Arabic alphabet. The corresponding treatments are often used by *sheikhs* in the state of purity (*wudû*) in Sufi medicine. If he needs a remedy for a specific disease, he creates a recipe consisting of words or numbers which often are also assembled to a geometric structure. The letters of the Arabic alphabet are in conjunction with numerical values; therefore, each word also has a numerical meaning. For example, the Arabic word for **God**, **Allâh**, consists of four letters: *alif, lam, lam* and *ha* and has the numerical value 66. Similarly, Quran verses have certain numerical values. The produced formula may now be used in different ways. For example, it is written, washed off, and drunk with plant color (e. g. saffron). Or it is attached to the affected part of the body. For the Sufi, the healing effect neither comes from the paper nor from the numbers or symbols. He exclusively attributes it to his Creator who invented these mental cures, made them available, and gave the permission for using them. Therefore, these cures are also referred to as „gracious prescriptions".

يا هو	يا هو	يا هو	يا هو
يا هو	يا هو	يا هو	يا هو
يا هو	يا هو	يا هو	يا هو
يا هو	يا هو	يا هو	يا هو

A protection *Ta`wîdh* against the evil eye and Djinns, which is attached to the clothes.

20

The traditional fasting

Fasting is part of the Sufi health program and one of the five pillars of Islam at the same time. *Ramadan* is the traditional fasting month of Sufis and Muslims. During this time, the original Holy Scriptures were revealed, including the Holy Quran. The duration of this fasting extends from sunrise to sunset. Meanwhile, the fasting person refrains from food, drink, tobacco use, and sexual intercourse. He should also, if possible, refrain from negative thinking, disputes, and other negative behaviors. This traditional fasting should not be seen in isolation. Additionally, the fasting believer prays and makes the prayer movements. In this way, he benefits from an additional blessing which gives him the necessary strength for fasting. In the case of „David' fasting", which traces back to the Prophet *David*, fasting is practiced every second day. The Prophet *Muhammad* – peace and blessings be upon Him – practiced it.

The purpose of fasting is to clean the body, spirit, and soul, it creates more sensitivity and receptivity to spiritual perception. It can also give an understanding of the knowledge and experience of the Divine. Furthermore, fasting strengthens the willpower. During this time, the body and its functions may rest and can revive and heal. Every fasting is a healing cure if it leads to better health and well-being. Numerous positive health characteristics are medically and scientifically proven, for example, in cases of overweight, arthrosis, arthritis, Alzheimer's, depressions, cancer, and rheumatism.

With their lack of knowledge, critics of the *Ramadan* claim that the Muslim fasting cannot be healthy, particularly because no liquid is taken in „such a long time". However, a healthy person is quite capable of doing without not only solid food, but also without fluid from sunrise to sunset. What is one day of this fasting (no more than about 20 hours, which is the case around the summer solstice)? Quite the contrary: researchers of the University of Southern California in Los Angeles have recently found out that regular, longer fasting does not only protect from damages to the immune system, but also supports its regeneration, indeed, can even generate a completely new immune system.

And here is a medical confirmation of the positive effects in the case of fluid removal: In his book *„Der Islam ist die heilende Medizin"* – *„ Islam is the healing medicine"* (publishing house Re Di Roma), the Syrian physician Dr. *Mohammad Omar Athai* writes: *„ ... water is not only important for the healthy and normal cells, but it also forms the most important basis for the existence of this dangerous ‚metabolic waste' that tries to ‚suffocate' the tissue. Only a consistent removal of water by fasting makes these harmful substances break apart and cleans the body so that the water can unfold its physiological task in clean tissue. ..."*

If you have no experience with fasting yet, you should seek advice and support by an experienced teacher, therapist, or doctor. In the event of existing diseases, fasting should only be (if at all) performed when monitored by a physician.

21

Sufis and their healing music

> *Whoever knows the secret of the sounds, knows the mystery of the universe.*
> Hazrat Inayat Khan

Sufis love and care for music. For them, it is nourishment for body, spirit, and soul. Among them, there are many excellent and famous musicians like *Nusrat Fateh Ali Khan, Abida Parveen, Shafqat Ali Khan, Omar Faruk Tekbilek, and others*. Especially using music as a medium and path of mystical experiences is of invaluable significance. Sufi music is of beneficial und healing nature. *Hazrat Inayat Khan*, a gifted musician himself, says: „Music is the best way to awaken the soul. There is no better one. Music is the shortest and most direct way to **God**.‟

Everything in the universe vibrates and chimes, has its own frequency, and penetrates itself constantly. When we understand and internalize that, phenomena like miracles and cures that are triggered by sound and music will be more understandable for us. These can certainly have different results, appear beneficial or destructive. The Indian musician *Tansen* is said to have been able to even light a fire through his sitars, playing at a certain time of day with a specific *raga*. Today, we also discover the great healing power of singing and sound, particularly with old instruments like sitar, flutes, drums, singing bowls, energy chimes etc. The music therapy is now an accepted therapy branch and is successfully used in education, psychology, and medicine. Sufis work a lot with the healing power of sound and tone. Already at an early stage, the people of Central Asia developed a music therapy which assumes that specific tone sequences have a healing effect on certain organs and body zones of the human being. We have to think of the spiritual music-making, singing, and reciting *Mantras* as a massaging of the body cells. The tone sequences used for this purpose are called *maqamat*; they are the equivalents to the Indian ragas or to the church tonal modes. In oriental music, we find a variety of *maqamat,* for example, from the pentatonic whose scale is not only considered as musical scale of peace and healing by the primitive people. Pentatonic melodies can also particularly be found in our children's songs and are used in music therapy. The doctor, shaman, musicologist, and Sufi sheikh *Orüc Güvenc,* founder of the school of ancient oriental music and art therapy (now: Institute for Ethno-Music Therapy), is one of the pioneers in this research area. He investigated the ancient knowledge of *maqamat* and uses it successfully. Sufis have developed an extremely differentiated way of singing and making music. They do not make music in a conventional manner with entertaining or soothing character. The chiming and singing takes place in meditation and often leads to a trance-like state. However, music always remains worship for the Sufi.

22

Sacred dances

Semâ, the wonderful whirling dance of the dervishes

The original Semâ ritual, the whirling dance of the dervishes, traces back to both the Persian poet Rumi and to Turkish customs. This festivity presents the spiritual journey of the human being, his orientation towards the truth and the divine, his ascent to heaven. The whirling dervishes (Semazen) take part with all their dedication and love. They whirl to the enchanting subtle Sufi music, played with exotic instruments and accompanied by virtuoso chants. In this ritual, the men with long white dresses and high felt hats do not only turn around on their own axis, but also circle around their sheikh standing in the middle - and this with closed eyes (!), sometimes for hours. In doing so, the dervishes always have absolute control of their body. They see Semâ as a way that promotes the inner development and the perception, frees the soul, and creates a connection to the divine. The authentic Semâ whirling dance is not that easy to learn and needs an intensive basic training under the guidance and supervision of an authorized teacher in the first place. The whirling itself, combined with Zikr and prayer, is a spiritual act. Many Sufis also practice a simple whirling dance, like little children do. But this whirling also needs constant control. The whirling has excellent health-promoting effects, activates the heart and circulation and all the organs.

Dances of Universal Peace

Apart from the traditional *Semâ* ritual, there are also Sufi orders and groups that practice traditional and self-created dances.

At the end of the sixties, *Samuel L. Lewis* (disciple of *Ruth St. Denis* and *Hazrat Inayat Khan*) started the „*Dances of Universal Peace*" in San Francisco. He created a sacred group dance which was accessible for all people due to its simplicity. In a wonderful combination of body and breath awareness with voice work, it has a healing effect on the body, spirit, and soul of people. During the hippie era, *Samuel L. Lewis* worked with young drug addicts. His work includes about 50 dances and experimental walking practices. In 1983, some of his disciples founded the „Peace Works International Center for the Dances of Universal Peace", a non-profit organization. Training programs are being offered worldwide. Meanwhile, there are more than 400 Dances of Universal Peace.

www.dancesofuniversalpeace.org

23

A healing ritual

The following ritual is a special healing ritual and for me personally, it has a particular significance: it was during the birth of my daughter *Malika Safina*. Complications of childbirth arose, her mother's blood flow was streaming constantly and if nothing significant happened, she was in danger of bleeding to death. I started to sing „Ya Shâfi, ya Kâfi", with a fervent voice and from the bottom of my heart, again and again. After about a quarter of an hour, the blood flow ran dry. We don't know whether mother and/or child would still be alive without this ritual, or rather without the help of **Allâh**, the All-Healing. Thanks be to Him! Al-HamdulilLâh! *Ya Schâfi, ya Kâfi!*

> **Healing ritual „Ya Shâfi, ya Kâfi"**
>
> *Ya Shâfi* means: „O You, Who You heal", and *Ya Kâfi*: „O You, Who You are able to do everything". With these two *Waza'if*, we call for the help and healing power of **God**. Here, they are always spoken or sung alternately, combined with the following movements:
>
> The participants stand in a circle. The person to be healed sits on a chair in the middle.
>
> The ritual starts with an invocation.
>
> In *„Ya Shâfi"*, the participants lift their arms upwards in a receiving manner and thus ask for the healing power of God. In *„Ya Kâfi"*, they help to

„transport" this power downwards and spread their arms out over the person to be healed. It is important that singing and movements are performed as evenly, calmly, and harmoniously as possible.

The teacher or leader of the group gives the sign for the next participant to come in the middle.

You can find the melodies or notes for „Ya Schâfi, ya Kâfi" also in the SUFI SONGBOOK (sol music). See also page 90.

At my events, I also use water that was spoken upon with Quran verses and is drunk by the participants at the end of the above ritual. In the next chapter, you will learn how this water is produced.

24

The healing water

> ... and we send down water from heaven according to the right measure, and we let it infiltrate into the soil. And we certainly have the power to take it away ...
> Holy Quran, Sura al-Mu´minun (the believers), Sura 23:18

> ... in other words: but consider, if the water of your wells and sources runs dry, who could supply you with fresh water? ...
> Holy Quran, Sura al-Mulk (The Kingdom), Sura 67:30

Water is our basis of life, we are not able to live without water. It is a great, wonderful grace of God. It symbolizes His mercy, wisdom, and infinity. God is the true source of life.

Naturally, pure water has a thirst-quenching, cleaning, and healing effect. It can have a powerful healing effect like the already mentioned water from the *Zamzam* source in the forecourt of the *Ka'aba* in Mekka. However, sources in other parts of the world also brought many blessings to people. Washings and water rituals are of importance in all spiritual traditions and religions. With the *Wudû´* ritual, the Muslim cleans himself with water at least five times a day.

By the way, did you know that our body only needs water to drink and as hydration? No fruit juice, no lemonade, no cola, or other beverages? Yes, our body contents itself „only" with water. How wonderful! Al-Hamduli**Llâh**!

In Ayurveda, it is a tradition to drink warm or hot water, which has extremely health-promoting effects.

Instruction for the manufacture of a healing water:

Here is the instruction for the manufacture of a healing water, which a fellow Sheikh of the *Naqschibandi* Sufi order gave us*:

- First, the speaking person performs *Wudû´*.
- This is followed by blessings *(Medet)* upon the prophets and the Sufi sheikhs.
- After that, the person concerned speaks the *Niyyah* with the words: „O **Allâh**, I intend to produce a healing water for .... (concerned person to be healed).
- Now the following prayers or Suras are spoken upon the water. A large bowl made of glass (no metal object!) is used for this purpose:

  4times **al-Fatiha,**
  7times **Ayat al-Kursi,**
  13times **Qulhu Allâhu ahad**
  then follows **Subhana rabbika ...**

*The speaking upon the water should be carried out by a competent, good person and sincere practitioner of Islam, who can recite the Holy Quran in a reading as authentic as possible. This person should also be in a healthy state at the time of the speaking upon and be well prepared in *Wudu* and for the ritual.

25

Sufis and humour

Sufis are funny, happy people and known for their witty, subtle humor. Their stories are teaching stories and have therapeutic effects. There are myriads of funny tales of *Mulla Nasrudin*, the oriental fools figure, the „Till Eulenspiegel of the Sufis", so to speak. Each of his stories, which were published in numerous books, show us an aspect of Sufism and can be seen as a mini-teaching. Each story, as the saying goes, has at least seven skins like an onion, accordingly, seven psychological teachings that have to be found out.

Nasrudin and the „deep-rooted pain"

Mulla Nasrudin rode with his donkey to a neighboring country to see the most sought-after psychiatrist there. „You must help me, I have a big problem!" Nasrudin urged. „What is the problem?" the psychiatrist asked. „Again and again, I feel a sharp, deep-rooted pain while walking," Nasrudin replied. They talked for quite a while, then the therapist diagnosed: „Your problem is that you hate your mother. Go home and come back tomorrow." Nasrudin was very impressed and due to his naivety, he went straight up to his mother. When he told her what the psychiatrist said to him, she fetched a big stick and hit him with it. Thereupon, Nasrudin went to his wife and cried on her shoulder. And she said: „Sometimes, your mother has quite good ideas!" and also hit him. The next day, Nasrudin went to the psychiatrist again and told him about the reactions of his mother and his wife. „Well, that is interesting! Now you also suffer from the delusion that everybody is hitting you. Come back again tomorrow." Finally, Nasrudin went to his daughter and told her everything, to which she replied: „I will not hit you, but let me give you a piece of advice: In the future, it would be better to walk behind your donkey and not in front of him. Because when you walk around with him deep in thought, he always bites deeply and firmly into your posterior ..."

Now it is up to the dear reader to guess the seven psychological levels (and also the errors in reasoning in the story ...) Have fun in doing so!

A small Sufi glossary

Al-asma' al-husna = the beautiful names of God. In the Holy Quran, we know 99 names (see p.29). However, beyond that, there are others, partly hidden ...

Allâh (t) = God (namely, the One, not a specific one). The addition or rather the abbreviation **(t)** means *Ta'ala* and is added when mentioning **Allâh**: *Allâhu* Ta'ala = **Allâh**, the Sublime.

AstarchfiruLlâh = „I ask God for His forgiveness" or „*Allâh*, forgive me".

Attar = plant essence or oil.

Basmala = designation of the words *Bismi Llâh ir-Rahmân ir-Rahîem.*

Breathing word = a word created by *Yan d'Albert,* which is connected to a certain breath and meditation technique.

Chishti or **Chishtiyya =** Indian Sufi order, initiated by *Hazrat Khwaja Moinuddin Chishty.* Poetry, music, and healing work are important elements in the lives of *Chishtiyyas.*

Dhikr or **Dhikru'l-Lâh** = remembrance, remembering God, recitation of sacred formulas and divine names.

Djinn (pl. **djinns**) (Arab.: those in hiding) are neither angels nor humans. They are demons made of more finer stuff.

Du`a´ = invocation.

Fatiha, al- = the Opening. This is the first, most recited, and shortest Sura of the Holy Quran (see p. 33).

Hadith = notification, report, a message of acts and sayings of the Prophet *Muhammad* – peace and blessing upon him.

Hadra = presence, attendance; gathering of the dervishes combined with *Zikr* and ecstatic „dances" or rather movements.

Ka'aba (Arab.: cube) = the cube-like building standing in the forecourt of the mosque in Mecca.

86

Maqâm (pl.: **Maqamât** or **Maqâms**) = station, spiritual place, also tomb; in the Sufi tradition, a state of mystic grace or a certain stage of consciousness or of the soul (see p. 65). In oriental music, tone scales similar to *modes (church modes)* are also understood to be *Maqâms*.

Miswak = a wooden toothpick usually made from a twig of the pelu tree

Niyyah or **Nyyat** = intention, formal declaration to do something.

Ramadan = Islamic month of fasting. In these days, God revealed the Holy Scriptures, also including the Holy Quran.

Salat = ritual prayer of the Muslims.

Schahada or **Shahada** = confession of faith and testimony of the Muslims. Designation for the words „*Ashadu an la ilaha illa Llâh, wa ashadu anna Muhammadan `abduhu wa rasuluh* = I testify that there is no God but **Allâh**, and I testify that Muhammad is His servant and messenger.

Sheikh (spelling also **Scheikh, Shaikh** or **Schech**) = word for word: old man; leader; also, a designation for a teacher, scholar, originally leader of a tribe (female equivalent: **Sheikha, Scheikha, Shaika, Schecha**).

Tariqa (pl: **Turuq**) = way, method, order, brotherhood or sisterhood or one of the four stages of Sufi-mystic experience and development.

Ta`wîdh = formula or amulet which contains verses from the Holy Quran, similarly, often also numbers.

Tesbih or **Tasbih** = common prayer chain in Islam, similar to a mala or a rosary. The word also means: praise of God.

Wazifa (pl.: **Waza´if** or **Wazifas**) = sacred words or mantras.

Wudû´ = washing or cleaning before the Muslim prayer *(Salat)* and other rituals *(Zikr,* etc.).

Books of Yan d'Albert (selection)

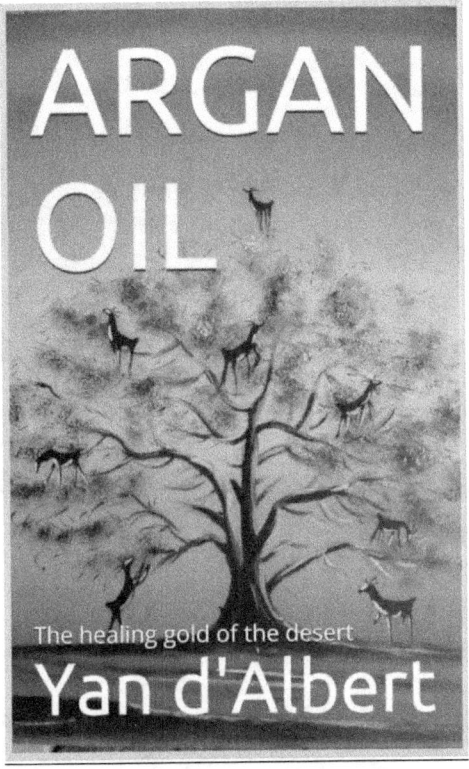

- ARGAN OIL - The wonderful healing power of desert gold, English edition (paperback, e-book, edition SOL 2014, available on Amazon)
- Publisher: Createspace Independent Publishing Platform (20 January 2016)
- Language: English
- Paperback: 26 pages
- ISBN-10: 1523614870
- ISBN-13: 978-1523614875

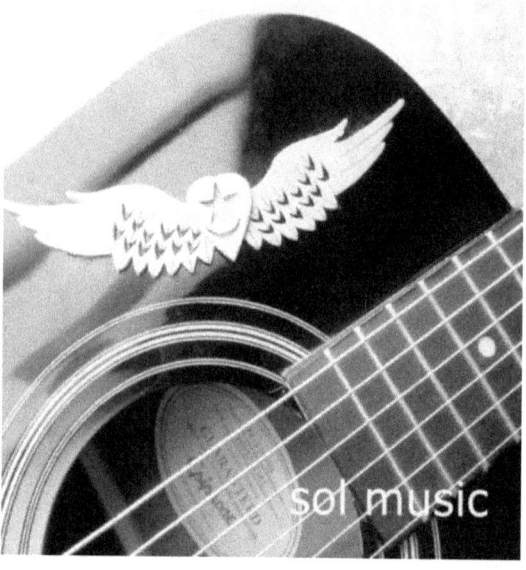

SUFI SONGBOOK

99 beautiful songs & mantras round the world

Yan d'Albert

sol music

The SUFI SONGBOOK is a unique collection of musical pearls. Written, arranged, produced and published by the author, musician and composer *Yan d'Albert* with much love and devotion. This songbook contains not only nasheeds, ilahis, songs, mantras & zikrs from the treasure chest of the Sufis but also from international traditions and religions who bear adequate spiritual reference e. g.: Folk songs, spirituals, psalms and more, 99 beautiful, inspiring and healing works.

(ring binder, paperback, e-book, sol music 2016, available on Amazon)

- Publisher; CreateSpace Independent Publishing Platform (18 December 2016)
- Language: English
- Paperback: 114 pages
- ISBN-10: 1540661628
- ISBN-13: 978-1540661623

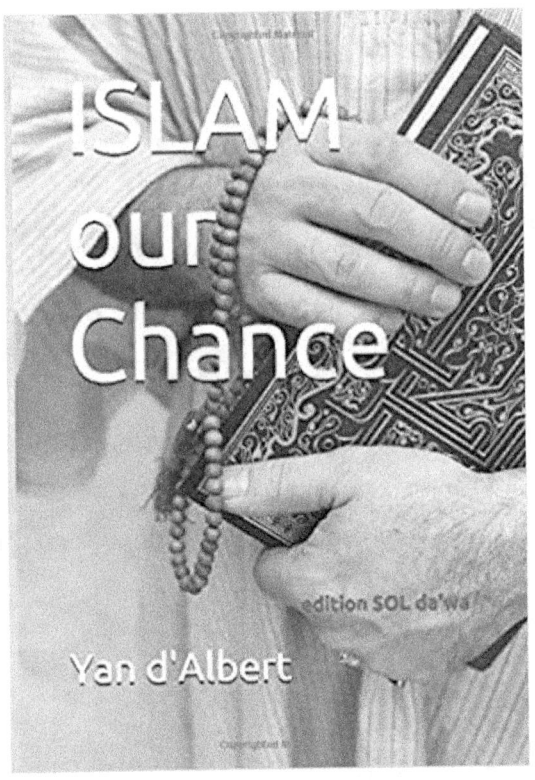

`Abd al-Malik Dildar Yan d'Albert (*1958), musician and author, converted to Islam in 1996. He has published numerous books, musical notes and CDs of Music, Sufism and Islam (e.g. the audio book and book "MUHAMMAD" – peace and blessings upon him - , the first authentic sira audio book in German language).

"ISLAM our Chance" is his personal heart project of da' wa, the invitation to Islam. Herin he tells, how ALLÂH, the Merciful, saved him with to books from "the descent into great success" as pop musician and how he found to Sufism and Islam. Despite all adversity he stood true to his music. Today he is a musician and music dealer much in demand, a happy husband and father. To be a Muslim means for him the greatest gift and the richest blessing of the One and Only, and the Holy Qur'an the most magnificent literary and musical work, and to practice Islam the fulfilment of his life.

For all persons interested in Islam and for future or new convertits. Also for Muslim siblings as a present to Non-Muslims. This little book is a real opportunity for spiritual seekers and truly a key to a fulfilled happy life, inscha **Allâh**.

(paperback, e-book, edition SOL da'wa, available on Amazon)

- Publisher: CreateSpace Independent Publishing Platform (11 July 2020)
- Language: English
- Paperback: 106 pages
- ISBN-13: 979-8644857555

www. Sufi healing sites

www.inayatihealingorder.org
www.dervish-healing-order.org
https://instituteofspiritualhealing.com
www.heilorden.de
www.sufiorden.at
www.sufismus.ch
www.sufihealingorderuk.org
www.sufiireland.com
www.inayatiorderfrance.org
www.sufi-danmark.dk
www.sufi.no

SUFI WAY OF HEART & HEALING /
MUSIKHAUS ALBERT
`Abd al-Malik Dildar Yan d'Albert
Odenthaler Str. 178
D-51467 Bergisch Gladbach (Germany)
Tel.: +49-22021085727
Mobil: +49-1775621773
yandalbert@t-online.de
musikhausalbert@t-online.de
www.yandalbert.de
www.musikhausalbert.de

Dear reader, Sisters & Brothers all over the world!

Thank you, that you have read this book. Don't hesitate to contact me, if you want.

Allâh, the All-Merciful, may guide and bless you for ever, inscha **Allâh!**

With all my heart

`Abd al-Malik Dildar Yan d'Albert

www.ingramcontent.com/pod-product-compliance
Lightning Source LLC
Chambersburg PA
CBHW062051280526
45788CB00003B/1187